GAO

Report to the Ranking Member, Subcommittee on Health, Committee on Ways and Means, House of Representatives

March 2012

MEDICARE SECONDARY PAYER

Additional Steps Are Needed to Improve Program Effectiveness for Non-Group Health Plans

I0428115

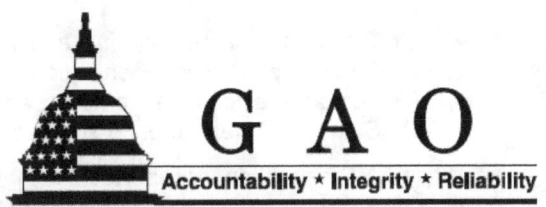

GAO

Accountability ★ Integrity ★ Reliability

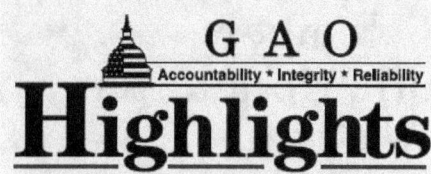

MEDICARE SECONDARY PAYER

Additional Steps Are Needed to Improve Program Effectiveness for Non-Group Health Plans

Highlights of GAO-12-333, a report to the Ranking Member, Subcommittee on Health, Committee on Ways and Means, House of Representatives

Why GAO Did This Study

The Centers for Medicare & Medicaid Services (CMS) is responsible for protecting Medicare's fiscal integrity. Medicare Secondary Payer (MSP) situations exist when Medicare is a secondary payer to other insurers, including non-group health plans (NGHP), which include auto or other liability insurance, no-fault insurance, and workers' compensation plans. CMS attempts to recover Medicare payments made that were the responsibility of NGHPs, but CMS has not always been aware of these MSP situations. In 2007, legislation added mandatory reporting requirements for NGHPs that should enable CMS to be aware of these situations. NGHPs reported concerns about the MSP process, and CMS delayed the start of mandatory reporting by NGHPs, in part because of these concerns. This report examines (1) how the initial implementation of mandatory reporting for NGHPs has affected the workload of and payments to MSP contractors, and Medicare savings, and (2) key challenges within the process for MSP situations involving NGHPs and the steps CMS is taking to address those challenges. GAO reviewed relevant MSP-related documents and data on MSP costs, workload, Medicare savings, and contractor performance. GAO also interviewed CMS officials, MSP contractor officials, and NGHP stakeholders.

What GAO Recommends

To improve the MSP program, GAO is making recommendations to improve the cost-effectiveness of recovery, decrease the reporting burden for NGHPs, and improve communications with NGHP stakeholders. CMS agreed with these recommendations.

View GAO-12-333. For more information, contact Kathleen M. King at (202) 512-7114 or kingk@gao.gov.

What GAO Found

During the initial implementation of mandatory reporting for non-group health plans (NGHP), the workloads of and Centers for Medicare & Medicaid Services (CMS) payments to Medicare Secondary Payer (MSP) contractors, and Medicare savings, all increased. From 2008 through 2011, the NGHP workloads of all three contractors CMS uses to implement the process for MSP situations—the Coordination of Benefits Contractor (COBC), the Medicare Secondary Payer Recovery Contractor (MSPRC), and the Workers' Compensation Review Contractor (WCRC)—increased to varying degrees. For example, from 2008 through 2011, the number of NGHP MSP situations voluntarily reported to the COBC increased from about 142,000 to about 392,000, the number of NGHP cases established by the MSPRC increased from about 238,000 to about 480,000, and the number of Medicare set-aside proposals submitted to the WCRC increased from about 20,000 to almost 29,000. From 2008 through 2011, the total CMS payments to the MSP contractors increased by about $21 million, and Medicare savings from known NGHP situations that CMS is able to track—including savings from claims denials and conditional payment recoveries—increased by about $124 million. The total impact of mandatory reporting on Medicare savings could take years to determine for various reasons, including that mandatory reporting is still being phased in.

Within the process for MSP situations involving NGHPs, GAO identified key challenges related to contractor performance, demand amounts, aspects of mandatory reporting, and CMS guidance and communication. CMS has addressed or is taking steps to address some, but not all, of these challenges.

- *Contractor performance.* Challenges related to the timeliness of the MSPRC and WCRC were identified, including significant increases in the time required to complete important tasks. CMS reported taking steps to address the challenges with each of these contractors' performance.

- *Demand and recovery issues.* Challenges were identified related to the timing of demand amounts, the cost-effectiveness of recovery efforts, and the amounts of Medicare demands from liability settlements. CMS reported taking steps to address some, but not all, of these challenges.

- *Mandatory reporting.* Key challenges were identified with certain aspects of mandatory reporting: determining whether individuals are Medicare beneficiaries, supplying diagnostic codes related to individuals' injuries, and reporting all liability settlement amounts. CMS reported taking steps to address some, but not all, of these challenges.

- *CMS guidance and communication.* Key challenges were identified related to CMS guidance and communication about the MSP process, guidance on Medicare set-aside arrangements, and beneficiary rights and responsibilities. CMS has taken few steps to address these challenges.

While CMS has taken, or reported it is in the process of taking, additional steps to address these key challenges, there are several areas related to the MSP program and process that still need improvement.

_____ United States Government Accountability Office

Contents

Figures

Abbreviations

CMS	Centers for Medicare & Medicaid Services
COBC	Coordination of Benefits Contractor
GHP	group health plan
HICN	Health Insurance Claim Number
ICD-9	International Classification of Diseases, Ninth Revision, Clinical Modification
MSA	Medicare set-aside arrangement
MSP	Medicare Secondary Payer
MSPRC	Medicare Secondary Payer Recovery Contractor
NGHP	non-group health plan
WCMSA	Workers' Compensation Medicare Set-Aside Arrangement
WCMSAP	Workers' Compensation Medicare Set-Aside Portal
WCRC	Workers' Compensation Review Contractor

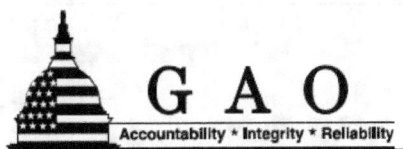
March 9, 2012

The Honorable Fortney Pete Stark
Ranking Member
Subcommittee on Health
Committee on Ways and Means
House of Representatives

Dear Mr. Stark:

In 2010, Medicare—the federal health insurance program that serves the nation's elderly and disabled—paid an estimated $509 billion to cover medical expenses for its 47 million beneficiaries.[1] While Medicare typically has primary payment responsibility for a Medicare beneficiary's medical expenses that are covered and otherwise reimbursable by Medicare, in some situations another insurer or insurers have the primary payment responsibility. In these situations, referred to as Medicare Secondary Payer (MSP) situations, Medicare is the secondary payer and is only responsible for paying for a beneficiary's Medicare-related health care costs that are not the responsibility of the primary insurer or insurers. The Centers for Medicare and Medicaid Services (CMS), an agency within the Department of Health and Human Services, is responsible for administering the Medicare program, including protecting its fiscal integrity. To safeguard funds, CMS must take steps to ensure that it pays only for those services that are the responsibility of the Medicare program.

Until 1980, Medicare was the primary payer in all situations involving Medicare beneficiaries except those covered by workers' compensation.[2] In 1980, Medicare became a secondary payer in all instances to non-group health plans (NGHP), which include auto or other liability

---

[1]Medicare is the federally financed health insurance program for persons age 65 or over, certain individuals with disabilities, and individuals with end-stage renal disease.

[2]Workers' compensation is a law or plan of the United States, or any state, that compensates employees who get sick because of their jobs or are injured on the job.

insurance, no-fault insurance, and workers' compensation plans.[3,4] For example, an NGHP is the primary payer for medical expenses related to injuries that a Medicare beneficiary sustains in an automobile accident (see fig. 1). Since 1982, Medicare has been a secondary payer to group health plans (GHP) in certain situations.[5]

Figure 1: A Medicare Secondary Payer Situation Involving an Auto Liability Insurer

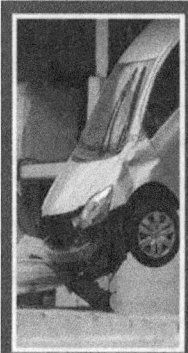

A Medicare beneficiary is injured in a car accident and goes to the hospital. The hospital bills Medicare, although the auto liability insurance company is responsible for paying for the beneficiary's treatment. Because the beneficiary has not yet reached a resolution with the auto liability insurance company, Medicare makes payments to the hospital for the care provided. Once the beneficiary receives a settlement from the auto liability insurance company, the Centers for Medicare & Medicaid Services seeks to recover the amount of Medicare's payments from the beneficiary.

Sources: GAO (text); Federal Emergency Management Agency/Casey Deshong (photograph).

When MSP situations have occurred, CMS has not always been notified that beneficiaries had other insurance that should be the primary payer. As a result, Medicare has paid for services that were the financial responsibility of another payer. Section 111 of the Medicare, Medicaid, and SCHIP Extension Act of 2007 added reporting requirements— referred to throughout this report as mandatory reporting—for NGHPs

---

[3]Omnibus Budget Reconciliation Act of 1980, Pub. L. No. 96-499, § 953, 94 Stat. 2599, 2647 (codified, as amended, at 42 U.S.C. § 1395y(b)(2)).

[4]Liability insurance is insurance that provides payment based on legal liability for injury or illness or damage to property. It includes, but is not limited to, automobile liability insurance, uninsured motorist insurance, underinsured motorist insurance, homeowners' liability insurance, malpractice insurance, product liability insurance, and general casualty insurance. No-fault insurance is insurance that pays for medical expenses for injuries sustained on the property or premises of the insured or in the use, occupancy, or operation of an automobile, regardless of who may have been responsible for causing the accident. 42 C.F.R. § 411.50(b).

[5]Tax Equity and Fiscal Responsibility Act of 1982, Pub. L. No. 97-248, § 116(b), 96 Stat. 324, 353. Although persons age 65 or older and persons under age 65 with certain disabilities are eligible for Medicare coverage, some may be employed and may receive health insurance coverage through an employer-sponsored GHP.

and GHPs with respect to MSP situations that should enable CMS to be aware of MSP situations.[6] Specifically, with mandatory reporting, CMS should be able to identify which payments made by Medicare should be recovered because another payer had primary payment responsibility and situations in which CMS should avoid making payments when another payer should be primary. Section 111 also included penalties for noncompliance with mandatory reporting ($1,000 fine per day of noncompliance per claimant). The Congressional Budget Office estimated that these provisions for NGHPs and GHPs would save Medicare $1.1 billion over 10 years in payments that could be recovered or avoided by Medicare.

Section 111 added mandatory reporting but did not eliminate or change any existing MSP laws or regulations. Prior to mandatory reporting, NGHPs and GHPs involved in MSP situations already had an obligation to notify and repay Medicare when they determined that Medicare should not have paid first. Likewise, Medicare beneficiaries had an obligation to take whatever actions were necessary to obtain any payment that could be reasonably expected from an NGHP or GHP and to cooperate with CMS in any action CMS took to recover payments Medicare had made. These obligations remain, although prior to mandatory reporting the parties involved in MSP situations may not have always complied with them. For example, prior to mandatory reporting, absent CMS being notified about an MSP situation and any specific correspondence from CMS to the beneficiary about MSP obligations, a beneficiary might not have been aware of any responsibility to repay Medicare for the related medical expenses.

MSP mandatory reporting has not been fully implemented. GHPs were required to begin reporting in January 2009. While NGHPs were scheduled to begin mandatory reporting in July 2009, CMS delayed this deadline several times, in part because of concerns raised by the insurance industry. Certain NGHPs, including workers' compensation and no-fault insurers, were required to begin reporting in January 2011. Other

---

[6]Pub. L. No. 110-173, § 111, 121 Stat. 2492, 2497 (codified at 42 U.S.C. § 1395y(b)(7-8)).

NGHPs, including most liability insurers, were required to begin phased-in reporting in January 2012.[7]

NGHPs and beneficiary advocacy groups have reported concerns related to CMS's process for handling MSP situations involving NGHPs. These concerns include issues with communication, policies and procedures, obtaining timely information, and the performance of MSP contractors. For example, NGHPs have reported disagreements with CMS MSP policies. Some of these difficulties may be because some NGHPs are interacting with CMS for the first time. These concerns were highlighted during a June 22, 2011, hearing held by the Subcommittee on Oversight and Investigations, House Committee on Energy and Commerce, about making improvements to the MSP process.[8]

Because of the reported concerns, you asked us to examine the issues surrounding the process for MSP situations involving NGHPs. In this report, we (1) describe how the initial implementation of mandatory reporting for NGHPs has affected the workload of and payments to MSP contractors, and Medicare savings, and (2) examine key challenges within the process for MSP situations involving NGHPs and the steps CMS is taking to address these challenges.

To determine how the initial implementation of mandatory reporting for NGHPs has affected the workload of and payments to MSP contractors, and Medicare savings, we interviewed officials from CMS and the contractors it uses to implement the MSP process about the effect of the initial implementation of mandatory reporting.[9] We also obtained and examined documentation and data from CMS and its MSP contractors regarding the contractors' workloads and CMS payments to the contractors, as well as data on Medicare savings for fiscal years 2008 through 2011. We interviewed CMS and MSP contractor officials about

---

[7]As of January 1, 2012, liability insurers (including self-insurers), are required to report settlement, judgment, award, or other payment amounts that are over $100,000 and were paid on or after October 1, 2011. At several specified dates in subsequent years, the reporting thresholds are to be reduced, and as of January 1, 2015, all settlement, judgment, award, or other payment amounts are to be reported.

[8]*Protecting Medicare with Improvements to the Secondary Payer Regime*, 112th Cong. (2011).

[9]For the purposes of this report, we consider the timeframe for the initial implementation of mandatory reporting to be fiscal year 2008 through fiscal year 2011.

the data received to learn about data collection methods, quality control efforts, and any data limitations. We determined that the data were sufficiently reliable for use in this report. We also interviewed NGHP stakeholders, such as organizations representing insurance companies and attorneys, to obtain their perspectives on how the initial implementation of mandatory reporting has affected their interactions with CMS and its contractors on MSP issues.

To determine the key challenges within the process for MSP situations involving NGHPs, we interviewed officials from CMS, its MSP contractors, and NGHP stakeholders, such as organizations representing insurance companies, attorneys, and beneficiaries, to better understand the MSP program and the process for situations involving NGHPs and their perspectives on any challenges within the process. In order to further understand the reported challenges, we also reviewed relevant CMS documentation, including MSP regulations, manuals, and user guides; CMS and contractor MSP-related web pages; and articles and reports by NGHP stakeholders and government agencies. We aligned the key challenges identified through interviews with other evidence, such as data on contractor performance and guidelines established in our *Standards for Internal Control in the Federal Government*[10] and the related *Internal Control Management and Evaluation Tool*.[11] To examine any steps CMS was taking to address the challenges, we interviewed officials from CMS, the MSP contractors, and NGHP stakeholders, and reviewed CMS and MSP contractor documents and websites.

We conducted this performance audit from February 2011 through March 2012 in accordance with generally accepted government auditing standards. Those standards require that we plan and perform the audit to obtain sufficient, appropriate evidence to provide a reasonable basis for our findings and conclusions based on our audit objectives. We believe that the evidence obtained provides a reasonable basis for our findings and conclusions based on our audit objectives.

---

[10]GAO, *Standards for Internal Control in the Federal Government*, GAO/AIMD-00-21.3.1 (Washington, D.C.: November 1999). Internal control is synonymous with management control and comprises the plans, methods, and procedures used to meet missions, goals, and objectives.

[11]GAO, *Internal Control Management and Evaluation Tool*, GAO-01-1008G (Washington, D.C.: August 2001).

Background

Medicare's payments in MSP situations can vary depending on the circumstances of the situation. CMS oversees all MSP activities and administers the MSP program, with contractors performing most of CMS's administrative activities within the process for MSP situations involving NGHPs. The process for MSP situations that involve NGHPs generally includes five basic components—notification, negotiation, resolution, mandatory reporting, and recovery.

Medicare Payments in MSP Situations Involving NGHPs

Medicare payments can vary in different MSP situations. In most MSP situations involving NGHPs, Medicare will pay initially for medical treatment related to the incident and later seek to recover those payments. When CMS is notified that an MSP situation exists in which an NGHP has accepted primary responsibility for ongoing medical services, Medicare will start denying the related claims. However, more commonly, CMS is notified about a potential MSP situation that is not yet resolved, and Medicare continues to make payments until the situation is resolved and there is a settlement, judgment, award, or other payment. Medicare does this to ensure that the beneficiary has access to needed medical services in a timely manner. CMS refers to any payments made by Medicare for services where another payer has primary responsibility for payment as conditional payments.[12] Once a resolution is reached between the beneficiary and the NGHP, Medicare will seek to recover any conditional payments made.

To help prevent Medicare from making future payments related to MSP situations involving NGHPs, when an individual is expected to have future medical expenses (including Medicare-covered drug expenses) related to his/her accident, injury, or illness, CMS states that all parties involved in negotiating a resolution of those situations are responsible for protecting Medicare's interests. One way to accomplish this is through a Medicare set-aside arrangement (MSA)—a voluntary arrangement where a portion of the proceeds from a settlement are set aside to pay for all related future medical expenses that would otherwise be reimbursable by

---

[12]CMS is authorized to make conditional payments when a primary payer has not or cannot make payment promptly. Such payments are conditioned upon reimbursement to Medicare. 42 U.S.C. § 1395y(b)(2)(B). The payment must be repaid to Medicare when a settlement, judgment, award, or other payment is made to the beneficiary from the NGHP.

Medicare if Medicare were the primary payer.[13] Medicare does not make payments for medical expenses related to the MSP situation until the MSA funds are exhausted. While MSAs can be used in liability or no-fault situations, they are most common for workers' compensation situations, where they are known as Workers' Compensation Medicare Set-Aside Arrangements (WCMSA).

Roles of CMS and CMS Contractors in MSP Activities

CMS oversees all MSP activities and administers the MSP program, through activities such as developing program policy and guidance. In addition, CMS communicates to stakeholders—including NGHPs, beneficiaries, providers, and attorneys—about the MSP process, policies, and guidance. For example, CMS maintains websites related to parts of the MSP process, from which NGHPs and beneficiaries can obtain information about their respective responsibilities in MSP situations involving NGHPs. GAO has established guidelines on internal control that are relevant for federal agencies such as CMS. Internal control includes the components of an organization's management that provide reasonable assurance that certain objectives are being achieved, including effective communication with external stakeholders.[14]

Since 2006, CMS has had three contractors to perform most of its administrative activities within the MSP process: the Coordination of Benefits Contractor (COBC), the Medicare Secondary Payer Recovery Contractor (MSPRC), and the Workers' Compensation Review Contractor (WCRC). Current contractor responsibilities are as follows:

- *COBC*: The COBC collects, manages, and maintains information in the CMS data systems about other health insurance coverage for Medicare beneficiaries and initiates MSP claims investigations. The information the COBC collects is available to other CMS contractors.

- *MSPRC*: The MSPRC uses information updated by the COBC as well as information from CMS's data systems to identify and recover

---

[13]In situations where an MSA is used, the responsibility for managing the MSA funds is not established by CMS. Thus, an MSA can be managed by various parties, including the beneficiary or a third-party administrator, such as an attorney.

[14]See GAO/AIMD-00-21.3.1. This document discusses key characteristics of specific internal controls and their essential role in communications, including that effective communications should include information flowing down, across, and up the organization.

Medicare payments that should have been paid by another entity as primary payer. Once a resolution has been reached between the beneficiary, or other individuals authorized by the beneficiary, and the NGHP, the MSPRC calculates the final amount owed to Medicare and issues a demand letter to the beneficiary or other individual authorized by the beneficiary.[15]

- *WCRC*: The WCRC evaluates proposed WCMSA amounts and projects future medical expenses related to workers' compensation accident, injury, or illness situations that would otherwise be payable by Medicare. The WCRC generally only reviews proposed WCMSA amounts for current Medicare beneficiaries within certain thresholds, referred to as CMS workload review thresholds.[16] WCRC-recommended WCMSA amounts are forwarded to one of six CMS regional offices for final approval.[17]

Process for MSP Situations Involving NGHPs

The process for MSP situations that involve NGHPs generally includes five basic components—notification, negotiation, resolution, mandatory reporting, and recovery. However, the details of the process, and the administrative tasks that must be conducted, can vary depending on when in the process notification occurs, the type of insurance involved (liability, no-fault, or workers' compensation), and the type of resolution

---

[15]This assumes a resolution in which the Medicare beneficiary or someone on the beneficiary's behalf receives a settlement, judgment, award, or other payment from the NGHP.

[16]The WCRC reviews proposed WCMSA amounts for injured individuals whose total settlement amounts are valued greater than $25,000 if the situation involves a current Medicare beneficiary and greater than $250,000 in situations where there is a reasonable expectation that the injured individual will become a Medicare beneficiary within 30 months of the date of the settlement. The WCRC rejects ineligible submissions—those that do not meet the workload review thresholds, are not related to workers' compensation cases, or involve black lung disease, as the Federal Black Lung Program pays first for any health care for black lung disease covered under that program. For the purposes of this report, we refer to all submissions to the WCRC as WCMSA proposals, even though they include some ineligible submissions that do not pertain to workers' compensation situations.

[17]The six CMS regional offices that provide final approval of proposed WCMSA amounts are Boston, Chicago, Dallas, Philadelphia, San Francisco, and Seattle.

reached.[18] While the details vary by situation and the timing of notification may vary, in general, the process contains the following components:

- *Notification*: The COBC is notified that a beneficiary's accident, injury, or illness is an MSP situation and creates a record. Notification can come from various sources—including the beneficiary, an attorney, a physician, or the NGHP—and can occur at various times during the process for MSP situations involving NGHPs. While mandatory reporting requires NGHPs to report MSP resolutions to the COBC, NGHPs or other involved parties may also provide voluntary notification earlier in the process. For example, a beneficiary's attorney could provide notification of an MSP situation involving an NGHP shortly after an accident occurs. After notification of the MSP situation, Medicare usually continues to make conditional payments although it may begin denying claims. Once the record for an MSP situation is created by the COBC, the MSPRC issues an MSP rights and responsibilities letter to the beneficiary or the beneficiary's representative, such as an attorney, which explains the applicable MSP law and how MSP recovery works.

- *Negotiation*: Negotiation occurs between the NGHP and the injured beneficiary or the beneficiary's representative. The point in the process at which notification of a potential MSP situation is made can affect the number and amount of conditional payments made by Medicare as well as whether, and the extent to which, information on conditional payments is available during the negotiation.[19] For example, if CMS is notified about a potential MSP situation early in the process, the MSPRC can provide information about what it has identified as any related claims that have been paid by Medicare. This information may then be used during the negotiations. This information is provided in writing through a conditional payment letter. For workers' compensation situations that involve future medical expenses, the WCRC may be involved in reviewing proposed WCMSA amounts.

---

[18]Because this report is focused on MSP situations in which an NGHP is the primary payer, when a resolution is referenced throughout this report we assume an outcome between a Medicare beneficiary and an NGHP in which there is a settlement, judgment, award, or other payment.

[19]If an NGHP immediately agrees to assume ongoing responsibility for a beneficiary's medical expenses, current and future, then there may not be a negotiation component to the MSP process.

- *Resolution*: Resolution is reached between the beneficiary or the beneficiary's attorney and the NGHP. The type of resolution varies and can include the NGHP assuming ongoing responsibility for payment of medical claims related to the injury or illness, a lump sum payment, a Medicare set-aside arrangement, or a combination of any of these. The beneficiary or the beneficiary's representative submits the resolution information to the MSPRC. For resolutions that include a WCMSA, no payments are made by Medicare for medical expenses related to the workers' compensation injury or illness until the set-aside is exhausted. The administrator of the WCMSA, typically the beneficiary or the beneficiary's representative, must submit an annual accounting of the set-aside funds to the MSPRC.

- *Mandatory reporting*: The NGHP reports the resolution to the COBC. Regardless of whether notification of the MSP situation occurred earlier in the process, after a resolution is reached in which the Medicare beneficiary or someone on the beneficiary's behalf receives a settlement, judgment, award, or other payment from the NGHP, the NGHP is required to report information about the MSP situation and its resolution to the COBC under mandatory reporting. The data NGHPs are required to submit include information to identify the beneficiary; diagnosis codes for the injury, accident, or illness; information concerning the policy or insurer; information about the injured party's representative or attorney; and settlement or payment information.

- *Recovery*: The MSPRC seeks to recover Medicare's conditional payments that have been made. The MSPRC calculates the total amount owed to Medicare and issues a demand for payment—referred to as a demand letter. This letter is typically issued to the beneficiary or the beneficiary's representative. The MSPRC compares the resolution data reported by the NGHP under mandatory reporting to any resolution data submitted by the beneficiary, or the beneficiary's representative, to ensure that the resolution data match. Either payment is received and the case closed or a response is received challenging all or part of the demand. If no response is received, debt delinquent more than 180 days is referred to the Department of the Treasury for collection action. The beneficiary has the right to question, appeal,[20] or request a waiver of recovery of the amount demanded.[21]

Figures 2, 3, and 4 illustrate how the process could work for MSP situations that involve an auto liability insurer, a no-fault insurer, and a workers' compensation plan, respectively. In each case, the timing of notification and the parties involved in each step can vary.

---

[20]Medicare beneficiaries have administrative appeal rights with respect to an MSP recovery claim against them that include five levels. The first level of appeal is to a CMS contractor. The second level of appeal is to an independent contractor to review the decision made at the first level of appeal. The third level of appeal is to an administrative law judge and must meet a minimum monetary threshold. The fourth level of appeal is with the Departmental Appeals Board before the Medicare Appeals Council. The fifth level is with the federal district court and has a minimum monetary threshold.

[21]The debt is not referred to the Department of the Treasury if there is open correspondence related to the debt or if there is a pending appeal or waiver request.

Figure 2: Illustration of the Process for a Medicare Secondary Payer (MSP) Situation Involving an Auto Liability Insurer

A Medicare beneficiary is injured in a car accident and goes to the hospital. The hospital bills Medicare. Medicare pays the hospital.

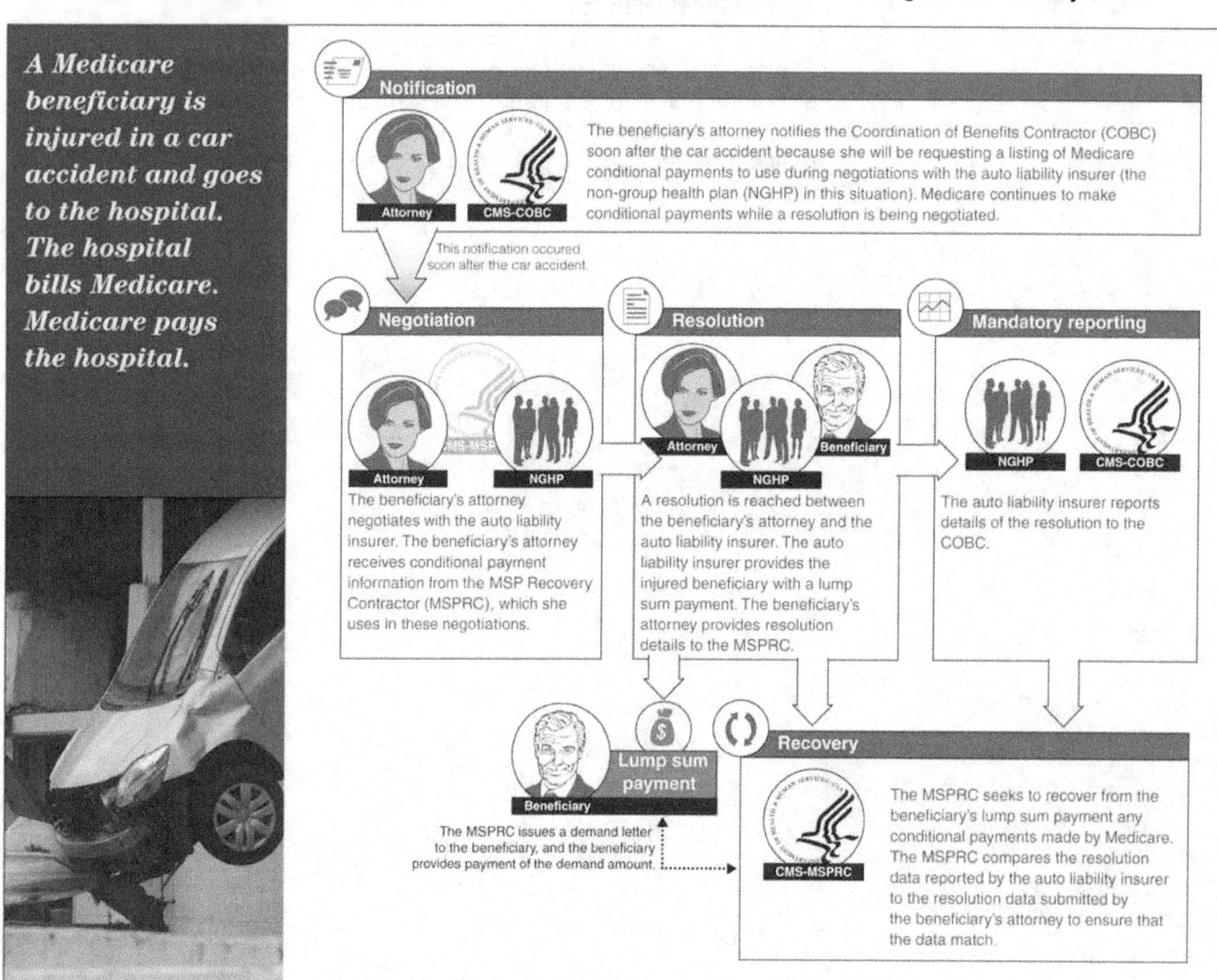

Notification

The beneficiary's attorney notifies the Coordination of Benefits Contractor (COBC) soon after the car accident because she will be requesting a listing of Medicare conditional payments to use during negotiations with the auto liability insurer (the non-group health plan (NGHP) in this situation). Medicare continues to make conditional payments while a resolution is being negotiated.

This notification occured soon after the car accident.

Negotiation

The beneficiary's attorney negotiates with the auto liability insurer. The beneficiary's attorney receives conditional payment information from the MSP Recovery Contractor (MSPRC), which she uses in these negotiations.

Resolution

A resolution is reached between the beneficiary's attorney and the auto liability insurer. The auto liability insurer provides the injured beneficiary with a lump sum payment. The beneficiary's attorney provides resolution details to the MSPRC.

Mandatory reporting

The auto liability insurer reports details of the resolution to the COBC.

Lump sum payment

The MSPRC issues a demand letter to the beneficiary, and the beneficiary provides payment of the demand amount.

Recovery

The MSPRC seeks to recover from the beneficiary's lump sum payment any conditional payments made by Medicare. The MSPRC compares the resolution data reported by the auto liability insurer to the resolution data submitted by the beneficiary's attorney to ensure that the data match.

Sources: GAO (process); Federal Emergency Management Agency/Casey Deshong (photograph); Art Explosion (illustrations).

Figure 3: Illustration of the Process for a Medicare Secondary Payer (MSP) Situation Involving a No-Fault Insurer

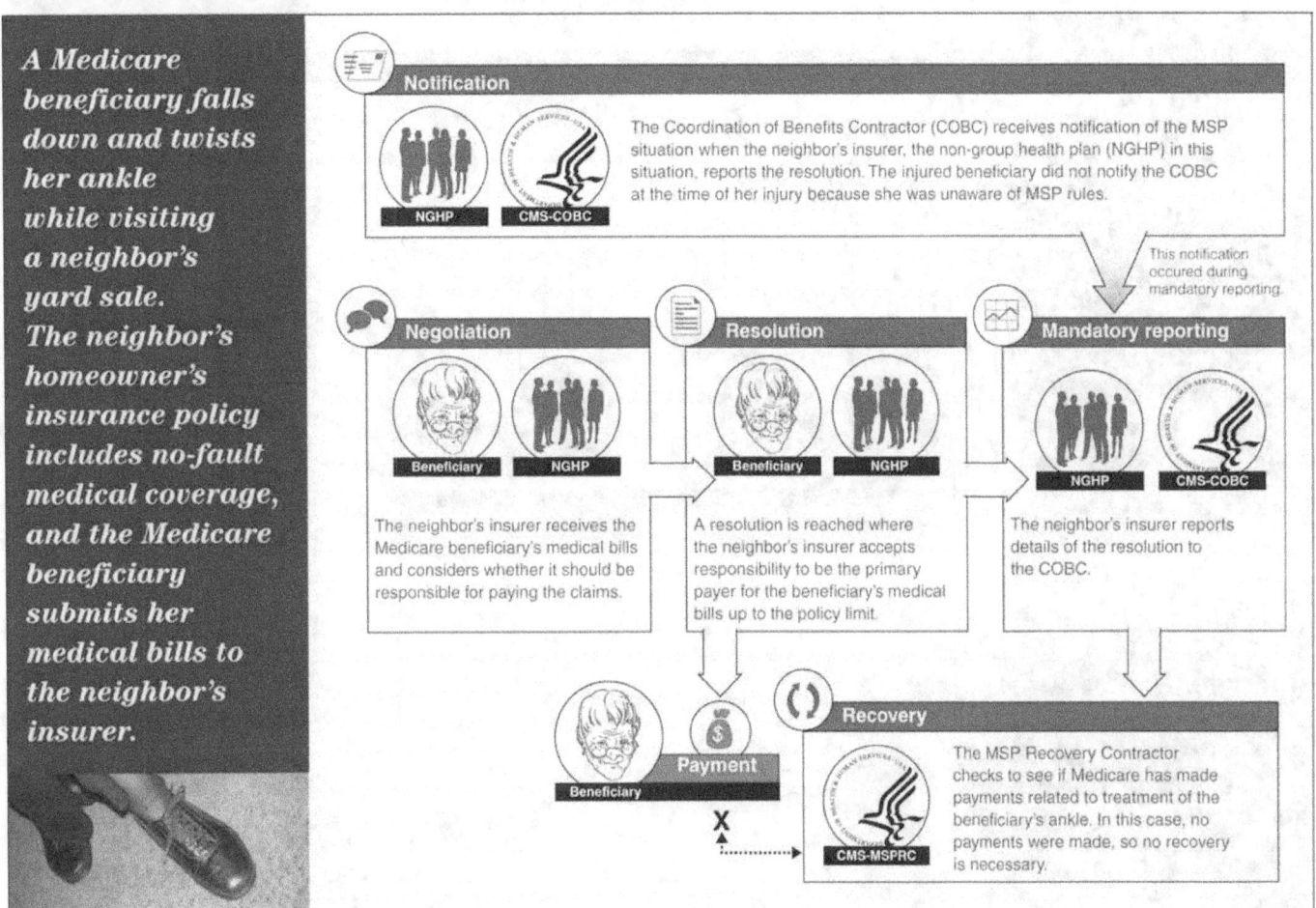

A Medicare beneficiary falls down and twists her ankle while visiting a neighbor's yard sale. The neighbor's homeowner's insurance policy includes no-fault medical coverage, and the Medicare beneficiary submits her medical bills to the neighbor's insurer.

Notification

NGHP   CMS-COBC

The Coordination of Benefits Contractor (COBC) receives notification of the MSP situation when the neighbor's insurer, the non-group health plan (NGHP) in this situation, reports the resolution. The injured beneficiary did not notify the COBC at the time of her injury because she was unaware of MSP rules.

This notification occured during mandatory reporting.

Negotiation

Beneficiary   NGHP

The neighbor's insurer receives the Medicare beneficiary's medical bills and considers whether it should be responsible for paying the claims.

Resolution

Beneficiary   NGHP

A resolution is reached where the neighbor's insurer accepts responsibility to be the primary payer for the beneficiary's medical bills up to the policy limit.

Mandatory reporting

NGHP   CMS-COBC

The neighbor's insurer reports details of the resolution to the COBC.

Payment

Beneficiary

X

Recovery

CMS-MSPRC

The MSP Recovery Contractor checks to see if Medicare has made payments related to treatment of the beneficiary's ankle. In this case, no payments were made, so no recovery is necessary.

Sources: GAO (process and photograph); Art Explosion (illustrations).

Figure 4: Illustration of the Process for a Medicare Secondary Payer (MSP) Situation Involving a Workers' Compensation Plan

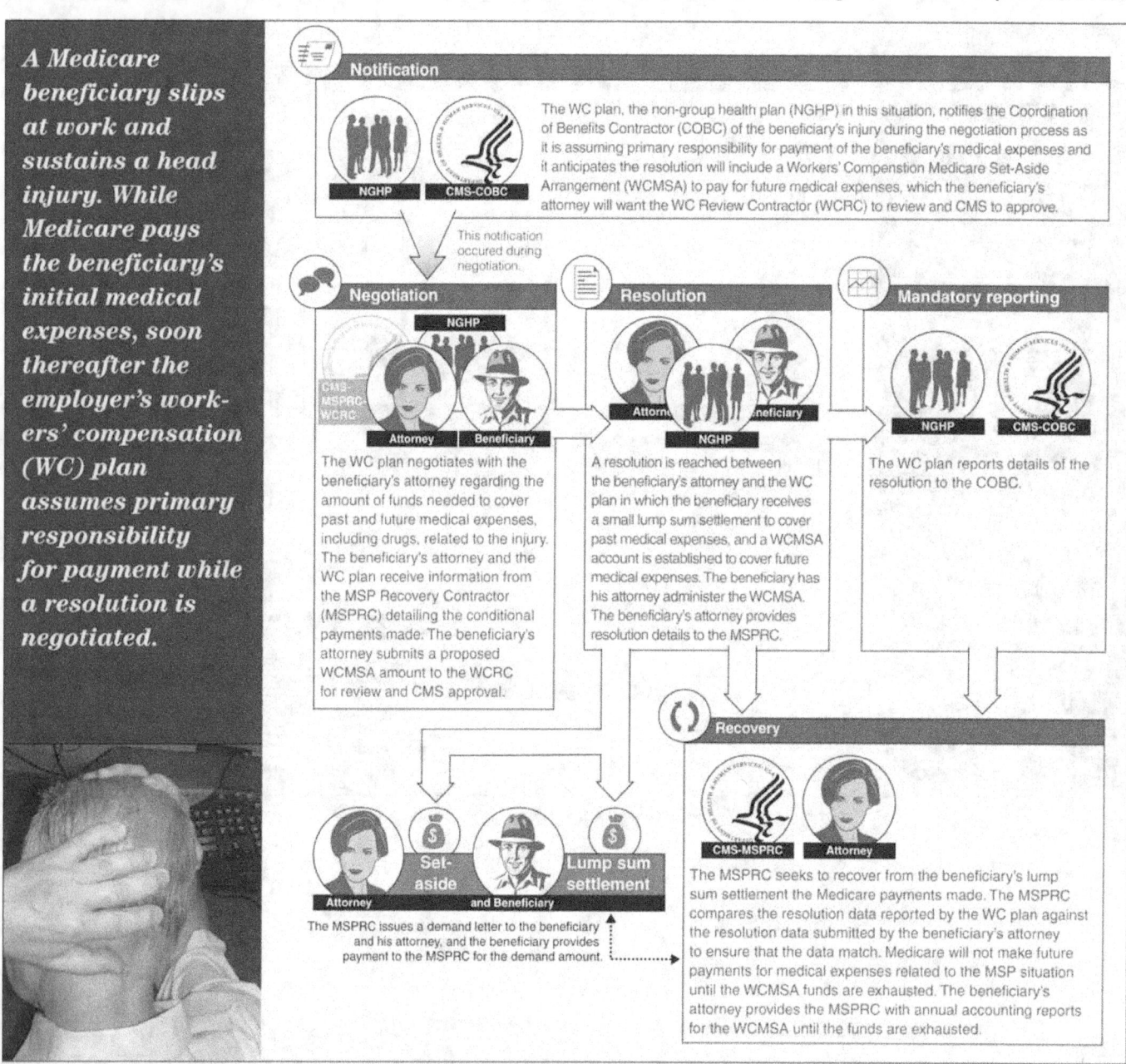

A Medicare beneficiary slips at work and sustains a head injury. While Medicare pays the beneficiary's initial medical expenses, soon thereafter the employer's workers' compensation (WC) plan assumes primary responsibility for payment while a resolution is negotiated.

Notification

The WC plan, the non-group health plan (NGHP) in this situation, notifies the Coordination of Benefits Contractor (COBC) of the beneficiary's injury during the negotiation process as it is assuming primary responsibility for payment of the beneficiary's medical expenses and it anticipates the resolution will include a Workers' Compensation Medicare Set-Aside Arrangement (WCMSA) to pay for future medical expenses, which the beneficiary's attorney will want the WC Review Contractor (WCRC) to review and CMS to approve.

This notification occured during negotiation.

Negotiation

The WC plan negotiates with the beneficiary's attorney regarding the amount of funds needed to cover past and future medical expenses, including drugs, related to the injury. The beneficiary's attorney and the WC plan receive information from the MSP Recovery Contractor (MSPRC) detailing the conditional payments made. The beneficiary's attorney submits a proposed WCMSA amount to the WCRC for review and CMS approval.

Resolution

A resolution is reached between the beneficiary's attorney and the WC plan in which the beneficiary receives a small lump sum settlement to cover past medical expenses, and a WCMSA account is established to cover future medical expenses. The beneficiary has his attorney administer the WCMSA. The beneficiary's attorney provides resolution details to the MSPRC.

Mandatory reporting

The WC plan reports details of the resolution to the COBC.

The MSPRC issues a demand letter to the beneficiary and his attorney, and the beneficiary provides payment to the MSPRC for the demand amount.

Recovery

The MSPRC seeks to recover from the beneficiary's lump sum settlement the Medicare payments made. The MSPRC compares the resolution data reported by the WC plan against the resolution data submitted by the beneficiary's attorney to ensure that the data match. Medicare will not make future payments for medical expenses related to the MSP situation until the WCMSA funds are exhausted. The beneficiary's attorney provides the MSPRC with annual accounting reports for the WCMSA until the funds are exhausted.

Sources: GAO (process and photograph); Art Explosion (illustrations).

MSP Contractor Workloads, Payments, and Medicare Savings Increased during the Initial Implementation of Mandatory Reporting for NGHPs

During the initial implementation of mandatory reporting for NGHPs, the workloads of and CMS payments to MSP contractors, and Medicare savings, all increased. For example, since fiscal year 2008, CMS payments to the MSP contractors have increased by about $21 million while Medicare savings from NGHP MSP situations—including savings from claims denials and conditional payment recoveries—have increased by about $124 million. However, because mandatory reporting is still being phased in, particularly for most liability settlements, it is too soon to determine the full impact of its implementation.

MSP Contractors' NGHP Workload Increased during the Initial Implementation of Mandatory Reporting for NGHPs

CMS MSP contractors' NGHP workloads increased during the initial implementation of mandatory reporting, and workloads are expected to continue to increase as mandatory reporting is phased in. The NGHP workloads of all three MSP contractors increased to varying degrees during the initial implementation of mandatory reporting. For example, from fiscal year 2008 through fiscal year 2011, the number of MSP situations involving NGHPs that were voluntarily reported to the COBC increased by 176 percent and the number of WCMSAs submitted to the WCRC increased by 42 percent (see table 1). Although mandatory reporting for NGHPs did not begin to be phased in until January 1, 2011, CMS officials told us that the effects of the mandate began earlier as the voluntary reporting of MSP situations (by NGHPs, attorneys, or beneficiaries) increased after the law's passage in December 2007.

Table 1: Medicare Secondary Payer (MSP) Contractor Non-Group Health Plan (NGHP) Workload for Fiscal Years 2008 through 2011

MSP contractor workload measure	2008	2009	2010	2011	Percentage increase, 2008 to 2011
NGHP MSP situations voluntarily reported to the Coordination of Benefits Contractor	141,890	185,085	357,747	392,254	176
NGHP cases established by the MSP Recovery Contractor	238,293	260,912	413,090	480,188	102
Workers' Compensation Medicare Set-Aside Arrangement proposals[a] submitted to the Workers' Compensation Review Contractor	20,255	24,203	26,296	28,847	42

Source: GAO analysis of MSP contractor data

[a]These include all submissions to the Workers' Compensation Review Contractor, including any that are later determined to be inelig ble for review.

CMS officials told us they expect that the COBC's and MSPRC's workloads will continue to increase once mandatory reporting is phased in for most liability MSP situations. CMS officials and an NGHP stakeholder group both told us that many liability MSP situations were not reported to CMS prior to mandatory reporting. CMS officials could not estimate the extent of future increases because CMS has no reliable estimates on the actual number of liability cases that include MSP situations.

The increased number of WCMSA proposals submitted to the WCRC during the past 4 years may be due, in part, to the NGHP industry's increased submission of ineligible and $0 WCMSA proposals in reaction to mandatory reporting. While the number of WCMSA submissions increased by 42 percent from fiscal year 2008 through fiscal year 2011, some of these submissions were not eligible for WCRC review—for example, they did not meet the minimum reporting thresholds—and the number of ineligible WCMSA submissions has grown rapidly. Ineligible submissions increased by about 148 percent from 2008 through 2011, growing from about 4,500 ineligible submissions in 2008 to about 11,200 ineligible submissions in 2011. Although mandatory reporting did not add any new WCMSA requirements, a CMS official told us the NGHP industry may be submitting more WCMSA proposals that are not eligible for WCRC review because it wants documentation from CMS stating that a WCMSA did not meet CMS's review thresholds.

Similarly, although not directly related to any reporting requirements, WCRC officials said that they have also seen an increase in $0 WCMSA proposals. A workers' compensation plan may submit these proposals when a settlement amount meets the minimum thresholds and is eligible for WCRC review, but the plan is asserting that it does not have responsibility for paying the beneficiary's future medical expenses. WCRC officials told us that when an NGHP submits a $0 WCMSA proposal, it may be seeking CMS confirmation that it does not have responsibility for paying the beneficiary's future medical expenses.

CMS's Payments to MSP Contractors Increased during the Initial Implementation of Mandatory Reporting

The total amount of CMS payments to the MSP contractors increased during the initial implementation of mandatory reporting.[22] Total CMS payments to the MSP contractors in fiscal year 2011 were about $21 million higher than payments in fiscal year 2008 (see table 2). Payments for the MSPRC's services increased by the greatest amount over this period—increasing about $16 million from 2008 through 2011. While CMS's overall contractor payments increased during this time period, the percentage increases in payments to the COBC and MSPRC were substantially lower than the increases in their workloads (see table 3).

Table 2: Centers for Medicare & Medicaid Services (CMS) Payments to Medicare Secondary Payer (MSP) Contractors for Fiscal Years 2008 through 2011

	Fiscal year				Payments percentage increase, 2008 to 2011
	2008	2009	2010	2011	
Coordination of Benefits Contractor	$40,358,460	$41,794,506	$47,171,893	$41,999,996	4
MSP Recovery Contractor	42,014,107	63,070,146	53,205,744	58,130,229	38
Workers' Compensation Review Contractor	3,817,289	5,264,402	4,986,204	6,715,620	76
Total	**$86,189,856**	**$110,129,054**	**$105,363,841**	**$106,845,845**	**24**

Source: GAO summary of CMS data.

Notes: "Payment" amounts and percentages are based on the amounts CMS obligated for the MSP contractors each fiscal year. A CMS official stated that the obligated amounts are an accurate reflection of the CMS payments made in each fiscal year to each MSP contractor. Total payments to the Coordination of Benefits Contractor and the MSP Recovery Contractor include payments for activities related to group health plan and non-group health plan MSP situations.

[22]"Payment" amounts are based on the amounts CMS obligated for the MSP contracts each fiscal year. A CMS official stated that the obligated amounts are an accurate reflection of the CMS payments made in each fiscal year to each MSP contractor.

Table 3: Percentage Increases in Medicare Secondary Payer (MSP) Non-Group Health Plan (NGHP) Workloads and Centers for Medicare & Medicaid Services (CMS) Payments to MSP Contractors, Fiscal Years 2008 through 2011

	NGHP workload percentage increase	Total CMS payments to MSP contractors percentage increase
Coordination of Benefits Contractor[a]	176	4
MSP Recovery Contractor[b]	102	38
Workers' Compensation Review Contractor[c]	42	76

Source: GAO analysis of CMS and MSP contractor data.

Notes: "Payment" amounts and percentages are based on the amounts CMS obligated for the MSP contracts each fiscal year. A CMS official stated that the obligated amounts are an accurate reflection of the CMS payments made in each fiscal year to each MSP contractor. Total payments to the Coordination of Benefits Contractor and the MSP Recovery Contractor include payments for activities related to group health plan and NGHP MSP situations.

[a]The workload measure used to calculate the percentage increase was the number of NGHP MSP situations voluntarily reported to the Coordination of Benefits Contractor.

[b]The workload measure used to calculate the percentage increase was the number of NGHP cases established by the MSP Recovery Contractor.

[c]The workload measure used to calculate the percentage increase was the number of Workers' Compensation Medicare Set-Aside Arrangement proposals submitted to the Workers' Compensation Review Contractor. The workload measure also includes submitted proposals that the Workers' Compensation Review Contractor determined were ineligible for review.

In order to control costs and contractor workloads, CMS is taking steps to improve the overall efficiency of the MSP program. CMS officials told us that they intend to move the MSP program to more of a "self-service" model. In this model, NGHPs, attorneys, and beneficiaries could obtain or submit required information through contractor websites or contractor automated phone lines, rather than submitting information via mail or fax, or waiting to speak to a customer service representative, as has traditionally been the process. This may result in increased efficiencies in the MSP process, for example, by allowing both NGHP stakeholders and MSP contractors to receive necessary information more quickly. Officials estimated that these steps will be able to reduce the workload performed per case by the MSP contractors.

Medicare Savings Increased during the Initial Implementation of Mandatory Reporting, but the Total Impact on Savings Could Take Years to Determine

Medicare savings increased during the initial implementation of mandatory reporting for NGHPs, but an accurate estimate of savings could take years to determine because of the lag time between initial notification of MSP situations and recovery, the fact that not all reported situations result in recoveries, and the fact that mandatory reporting is still being phased in. MSP savings from known NGHP situations that CMS is able to track—including savings from claims denials and conditional payment recoveries—increased by about $124 million from fiscal year

2008 through fiscal year 2011. Savings attributable to liability insurance increased by the greatest amount during this time period, growing from about $342 million in fiscal year 2008 to about $448 million in fiscal year 2011. In addition to these savings, Medicare also avoids costs as a result of the use of MSAs. CMS only tracks cost-avoided savings attributable to approved WCMSA proposals, not other types of MSAs, and accounts for the savings by reporting the total WCMSA amounts approved each fiscal year.[23] These numbers therefore represent the maximum cost-avoided savings that could potentially be realized through these WCMSAs in the future. See table 4 for the total amount of MSP savings from NGHP situations and WCMSAs approved from fiscal year 2008 through fiscal year 2011. Because of a change in CMS policy implemented in 2009, it is unclear to what extent the increases in approved WCMSA amounts can be attributed to mandatory reporting.[24]

---

[23]While this does not accurately project the year in which the savings would actually be incurred, it does provide some additional information about the extent to which Medicare is getting cost-avoided savings through the WCMSA process. CMS is not able to track savings attributable to WCMSAs that are not submitted to, and approved by, CMS.

[24]In June of 2009, CMS began independently calculating expenses for prescription drug treatments included in WCMSA proposals. Prior to that, WCMSA submitters had been using their own calculations for prescription drug treatments, and the conventions used to establish these prices varied among the submitters.

Table 4: Medicare Savings from Medicare Secondary Payer (MSP) Situations Involving Non-Group Health Plans (NGHP) and Approved Workers Compensation Medicare Set-Aside Arrangement (WCMSA) Amounts, Fiscal Years 2008 through 2011

NGHP MSP situation savings[a]	2008	2009	2010	2011	Percentage increase, 2008 to 2011
Workers' compensation	$136,907,844	$107,201,462	$169,960,944	$142,736,039	4
No-fault insurance	258,728,298	248,181,610	326,282,034	271,117,941	5
Liability insurance	341,702,138	323,768,272	424,568,902	447,889,979	31
Total	**$737,338,280**	**$679,151,344**	**$920,811,880**	**$861,743,959**	**17**
Approved WCMSA amounts[b]	**$905,202,448**	**$1,125,261,415**	**$1,443,739,397**	**$1,102,662,414**	**22**

Source: GAO summary of CMS data.

[a]Savings attributable to MSP situations involving NGHPs were calculated by combining known, tracked savings from claims denials, recoveries, and CMS data matching activities to identify situations where another payer may be primary to Medicare and conducted with the Social Security Administration and Internal Revenue Service.

[b]The total approved WCMSA amounts include the total amounts approved in each fiscal year, and represent the maximum cost-avoided savings that could potentially be realized through these WCMSAs in the future. While this does not accurately project the year in which the savings would actually be avoided, it does provide some additional information about the extent to which Medicare is getting cost-avoided savings through the WCMSA process. CMS is not able to track savings attributable to WCMSAs that are not submitted to, and approved by, CMS.

While Medicare savings attributable to NGHP MSP situations have been increasing overall, it is too soon to determine the total impact that mandatory reporting will have on NGHP Medicare savings. Savings amounts have not increased as quickly as the overall increase in NGHP MSP situations reported to CMS. There are two reasons why this may be occurring. CMS officials told us that because it can take several years for a case involving an NGHP MSP situation to be resolved, there is a delay between when increases are seen in the number of new situations reported and when increases are seen in the amounts of demands and recoveries. Additionally, since there is not necessarily a recovery demand issued for every NGHP situation reported, an increase in the number of reported cases will not necessarily result in a corresponding increase in recoveries. These MSP situations represent cost-avoided savings, but CMS officials told us that to the extent that these situations are working appropriately and CMS is not receiving claims, they have no way of knowing the savings associated with these situations.

CMS Is Addressing Some but Not All of the Key Challenges We Identified within the Process for MSP Situations Involving NGHPs

Within the process for MSP situations involving NGHPs, we identified key challenges related to contractor performance, demand amounts, aspects of mandatory reporting, and CMS guidance and communication. CMS has addressed, or is taking steps to address some, but not all, of these challenges.

CMS Is Taking Steps to Address Challenges Related to MSPRC and WCRC Timeliness

Challenges related to the timeliness of the MSPRC and WCRC were identified, including recent significant increases in the time required to complete certain processes or tasks, and CMS reported taking steps to address the challenges with each of these contractors' performance.

MSPRC Performance

Problems related to the timeliness of the MSPRC have been identified, and several actions have been taken or are under way by CMS to address these problems. NGHPs and beneficiary advocates have cited performance problems with the MSPRC that include the length of time taken to answer phone calls and to issue demand letters after resolutions for an MSP situation were provided to the MSPRC. MSPRC data show that from fiscal year 2008 through fiscal year 2011 the average wait time for NGHP callers has increased from an average of less than 3 minutes to an average of more than 38 minutes. During that same period, the number of NGHP-related calls handled by the MSPRC's customer service representatives increased from about 550,000 in fiscal year 2008 to about 630,000 in fiscal year 2011, and the number of calls abandoned after 31 seconds or more increased from about 30,000 in fiscal year 2008 to about 220,000 in fiscal year 2011. CMS officials told us that while the MSPRC did not have a specific performance standard for average call wait times in its contract, they found the current average wait time of over 38 minutes for NGHP-related phone calls unacceptable.

In fiscal year 2011, the MSPRC averaged about 76 days to issue a demand letter when notice of settlement was the initial notification of the MSP situation to the MSPRC. If the MSPRC was aware of the MSP situation prior to receiving the notice of settlement, it averaged about 48 days to issue a demand letter. Delays in issuing demand letters could result in delays in distributing funds from MSP situation resolutions to beneficiaries. CMS officials stated that the agency has a performance standard stating that the issuance of a demand letter within 20 days is timely if the case was established prior to settlement and the initial conditional payment letter was issued.

CMS and MSPRC officials attributed some of the MSPRC's performance challenges to higher-than-expected workloads. MSPRC officials attributed their inability to keep up with increased call volumes to a lack of resources, stating that since the contract's inception they have not been adequately funded by CMS for their workloads. They stated that CMS has consistently underestimated the annual volume of calls the MSPRC would receive. CMS officials acknowledged that when the contract started in 2006, at which time the MSP recovery tasks were transitioned from CMS claims contractors to the MSPRC, CMS underestimated the MSPRC workload. Officials said that just when the MSPRC was close to catching up from that transition, mandatory reporting was announced, which created a new, additional workload.

CMS reported that the agency was taking several steps intended to address MSPRC performance challenges. For example, CMS did not renew the contract with the entity that served as the MSPRC since October 1, 2006, and is planning to make a significant change to its current MSP contracting structure by combining the functions of the current COBC and MSPRC. CMS intends to streamline the MSP data and debt collection processes for Medicare stakeholders by establishing a centralized coordination of benefits and MSP recovery organization. CMS reports that this approach will allow the agency to minimize duplicative activities that were previously performed by both the COBC and MSPRC, provide a single point of contact for internal and external stakeholders, and consolidate MSP responsibility under one umbrella. CMS is also working to develop a web-based MSPRC portal, which will enable beneficiaires and beneficiaries' representatives to, among other things, obtain information about their Medicare claim payments. Table 5 presents the steps CMS is taking to address MSPRC performance challenges and the anticipated results of taking these steps. Most of these steps were either implemented only recently or have not yet been implemented, therefore it is too soon to tell to what extent these functions currently performed by the MSPRC will improve as a result of these actions.

Table 5: Steps the Centers for Medicare & Medicaid Services (CMS) Is Taking to Address Medicare Secondary Payer Recovery Contractor (MSPRC) Performance Challenges and the Anticipated Results

Steps CMS is taking to address MSPRC performance challenges	Anticipated results
Establishing a centralized coordination of benefits and Medicare Secondary Payer (MSP) recovery organization	Provide greater efficiency and oversight by: minimizing duplicative activities previously performed by both the Coordination of Benefits Contractor (COBC) and MSPRC and provide a single point of contact for internal and external stakeholders.
Contracted with current COBC to serve as the new interim MSPRC contractor	Minimal disruption to the services provided to beneficiaries, attorneys, and non-group health plans (NGHP) while the details of the new combined COBC MSPRC contracts are worked out.
Self-service MSPRC phone line[a]	Reductions in call wait times.
Improvements to MSPRC processes	Improve the timely issuance of demand letters; the agency will continue to monitor these activities and make revisions as necessary.
Develop MSPRC web portal[b]	Reduce contractor workload and help relieve problems related to contractor responsiveness.

Source: GAO analysis.

[a]Through the self-service, automated phone line, stakeholders can obtain up-to-date conditional payment and demand amounts, as well as the dates the MSPRC issues letters.

[b]The web-based MSPRC portal, which CMS anticipates will be implemented in July 2012, will allow the beneficiary, or beneficiary's representative, to obtain information about Medicare's conditional payments and input information about disputed claims (claims that the beneficiary asserts are unrelated to the MSP situation).

WCRC Performance

The average processing time for the WCRC to review WCMSA proposals has increased significantly over the past year and a half, resulting in delays in the resolution of MSP cases, and several actions have been taken or are under way by CMS that are intended to reduce processing time. According to WCRC data, the average processing time for all cases increased from 22 days in April 2010 to 95 days in September 2011 (see fig. 5).[25] While the current WCRC contract does not include a performance standard related to the length of time for the WCRC to review submitted WCMSA proposals, WCRC officials told us they would like WCMSA reviews to be completed within 45 days. CMS and WCRC officials report that a number of factors contributed to the WCRC's review process taking longer, including increased workload. For example, while in fiscal year 2011 the WCRC contract estimated that the WCRC would

---

[25]These numbers do not include cases where the regional offices request the WCRC to conduct a re-review. CMS regional offices may, at their discretion, request that the WCRC perform a re-review of WCMSAs. This may occur if, for example, the regional office finds an error in the WCRC's original review, or if the WCMSA submitter provides additional information after the WCRC's review is complete that should have been considered during its initial review.

review 1,700 WCMSA proposals each month, the WCRC received an average of about 2,400 WCMSA proposals per month and was able to review an average of about 2,100 per month. As a result, a backlog grew. According to WCRC data, over the past several years, an increasing number of submitted WCMSA proposals were determined by the WCRC to be ineligible for review, meaning that more of the WCRC's time has been spent responding to ineligible proposals. Also, CMS reported that a change made to the data system used by the WCRC to process WCMSAs resulted in a decrease in system performance, which significantly increased review time from September 2010 through January 2011, adding to the backlog of WCMSA proposals to be reviewed.

Figure 5: Workers' Compensation Review Contractor (WCRC) Average Processing Time for Workers' Compensation Medicare Set-Aside Arrangement Proposals, April 2010 through September 2011

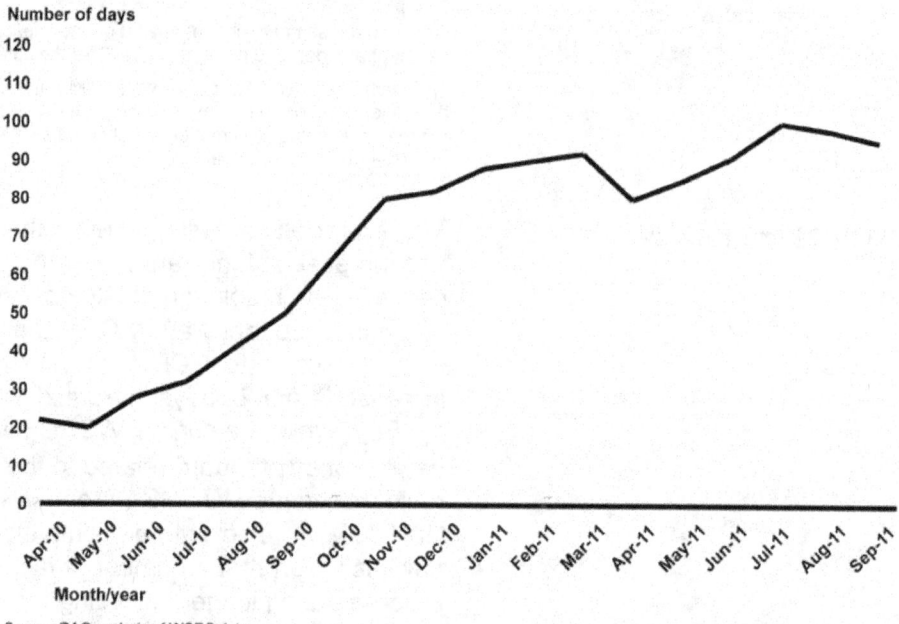

Source: GAO analysis of WCRC data.

Several actions have been taken or are under way by CMS to reduce the average processing time for WCMSA proposal review. For example, in fiscal year 2011 CMS provided the WCRC with additional funding that enabled the WCRC to authorize overtime for its employees to attempt to decrease the existing backlog of submitted WCMSA proposals. CMS is also currently in the process of awarding a new WCRC contract. According to CMS officials, the new contract provides for an increased estimated number of monthly WCMSA proposal reviews—increasing the number from 1,700 a month to from 2,000 to 2,500 a month. Additionally, CMS implemented a web-based portal—the WCMSA Portal (WCMSAP)—which is intended to improve the efficiency of the WCMSA submission process. The WCMSAP allows registered users, such as beneficiaries, attorneys, and insurance companies, to directly enter WCMSA case information electronically, upload documentation, and receive up-to-date case status information electronically. CMS conducted a pilot test with 10 WCMSA submitters that according to COBC officials, collectively represented 80 percent of all WCMSA submissions. We contacted the 10 WCMSA submitters that participated in the WCMSAP pilot, and they told us that the WCMSAP could improve the overall WCMSA submission and review process.[26] The WCMSAP became available for use by all WCMSA submitters on November 29, 2011. Finally, CMS hired a contractor to conduct an assessment of its WCMSA process, which could result in recommendations to address related policies and procedures, such as the average processing time. CMS officials told us that they expected to receive a draft of the contractor's report in March 2012, with a final report in June 2012.

CMS Is Taking Steps to Address Some of the Key Demand and Recovery Challenges We Identified

We identified three key challenges related to demand and recovery of MSP amounts. They include challenges related to the timing of the final demand amounts, the cost-effectiveness in recovery efforts, and the amounts demanded in liability settlements. CMS officials reported that the agency was taking steps to address some, but not all, of these challenges.

Timing of Final Demand Amount

Stakeholders, such as attorneys and NGHPs, reported that because CMS does not provide a final demand amount prior to a settlement, they have difficulty determining an appropriate settlement amount, which delays settlements. CMS is taking several steps to address this challenge. NGHP stakeholders reported that it would be helpful if CMS could calculate a final demand amount that can be provided to concerned parties prior to settlement, rather than after settlement. CMS officials stated, however, that they do not know what the final demand amount will be because Medicare continues to make conditional payments up to the

---

[26]CMS told us that WCMSA submitters will be able to continue to mail hard copies of WCMSA proposal submission documents to the COBC to process and forward to the WCRC for review even after the WCMSAP's implementation.

settlement date.[27] CMS officials also noted that during settlement negotiations, beneficiaries can view all their claims paid to date by Medicare on the MyMedicare.gov website.

CMS is taking steps that may improve NGHP stakeholders' ability to obtain or estimate Medicare's demand amount prior to settlement. For example, as of September 30, 2011, beneficiaries can obtain the latest issued Medicare conditional payment amounts through an automated, self-service feature of the MSPRC phone line. In November 2011, CMS implemented an option for beneficiaries to pay Medicare a fixed 25 percent of their settlement amount for certain liability situations involving a physical-trauma-based injury with settlement amounts of $5,000 or less.[28] In December 2011, CMS announced an option for beneficiaries, beginning in February 2012, to self-calculate conditional payment amounts for liability insurance MSP situations with settlement amounts of $25,000 or less that involve physical-trauma-based injuries.[29] The MSPRC will review the proposed self-calculated conditional payment amount and, if it finds the amount accurate, will respond with Medicare's final conditional payment amount within 60 days.

Recovery Cost-effectiveness

CMS has sometimes spent more in administrative costs attempting to recover certain conditional payment amounts than the demands are actually worth, but has recently implemented two initial recovery thresholds and may consider additional thresholds once it has had an opportunity to review 2012 data. NGHP stakeholders provided an example of a demand letter issued by the MSPRC for an amount of

---

[27]CMS does, however, have an alternate process it uses to calculate its recovery claim for certain situations which the agency refers to as global resolutions. In these cases, when CMS has determined it is cost effective to do so, CMS uses modeling to calculate Medicare's recovery claim for a group of Medicare beneficiaries. For example, officials said that this modeling might be used in the instance of a group of Medicare beneficiaries who were injured as a result of taking a particular prescription drug.

[28]The beneficiary must also elect this option prior to the MSPRC issuing a demand letter, and the beneficiary must not have received, and not expect to receive, any other settlements related to the incident.

[29]The beneficiary's date of incident must have occurred at least 6 months before the beneficiary or the beneficiary's representative submitted the proposed self-calculated conditional payment amount to the MSPRC. The beneficiary must also demonstrate that treatment has been completed and no further treatment is expected, and the beneficiary must settle within 60 days after the date of Medicare's response with the final conditional payment amount.

$1.59; one NGHP stakeholder noted seeing numerous examples of demand letters for amounts less than $5.00. MSPRC officials confirmed that they have traditionally pursued any recoveries the MSPRC was made aware of, regardless of the administrative costs to recover them. In 2004 we noted the importance of improving the cost-effectiveness of the MSP recovery process, and CMS concurred with our recommendations.[30] The cost-effectiveness of recovery has improved greatly. In 2004, we reported that CMS recovered only 38 cents for every dollar spent on recovery activities in fiscal year 2003, but in June 2011 CMS reported that MSP activities have provided an average rate of return on recoveries of $9.32 for each dollar spent since fiscal year 2008. NGHP stakeholders suggested that CMS should take an additional step to improve cost-effectiveness by setting a recovery threshold based on the settlement amount that would likely yield a recovery amount at or above CMS's cost to recover that money.

CMS has already implemented two initial recovery thresholds, and is currently reviewing and evaluating its costs and recovery data. CMS officials report that they are considering implementing additional, higher recovery thresholds, if appropriate, that balance protecting Medicare's interests and responding to the NGHP stakeholders' concerns. For example, on June 30, 2011, CMS instructed the MSPRC to cease issuing demands for amounts of $25 or less. CMS officials told us that the agency selected the $25 threshold based on provisions in the Federal Claims Collection Act and on the MSPRC's collection costs.[31] In addition, in September 2011 CMS announced that the agency would not act to recover certain liability settlements of $300 or less, based on a preliminary analysis of all NGHP recoveries, which determined that the MSPRC's average recovery cost per NGHP case was between $150 and

---

[30]See GAO, *Medicare Secondary Payer: Improvements Needed to Enhance Debt Recovery Process*, GAO-04-783 (Washington, D.C.: Aug. 20, 2004), 20-21.

[31]Among other things, the Federal Claims Collection Act permits the Secretary of Health and Human Services to end collection actions on certain claims when the cost of collecting such claims is likely to be more than the amount recovered. 31 U.S.C. § 3711(a)(3). *See also*, 31 C.F.R. §§ 903.1-903.5. Additionally, the MSP statutory provision provides for the waiver of conditional payment requirements, including repayment, when the Secretary determines that such a waiver is in the best interests of Medicare. 42 U.S.C. § 1395y(b)(2)(B)(v).

$200.[32] CMS officials report that the agency will consider establishing additional recovery thresholds for certain NGHP situations once officials have had a chance to review 2012 data, which will include information on some liability MSP situations.

Demand Amounts in Liability Settlements

NGHP stakeholders suggested that because CMS does not recognize the concept of proportionality in liability settlement situations a disproportionate share of liability settlement amounts may be paid to Medicare; however, CMS has a process that may sometimes address this challenge. The concept of proportionality in liability settlement amounts is relevant in situations when individuals and liability insurers agree to settle for less than the full amount of incurred expenses associated with the alleged incident, and therefore the amount of medical expenses to be reimbursed to an individual's health plan is proportionally reduced. NGHP stakeholders said that CMS does not recognize this concept for MSP situations and instead wants 100 percent reimbursement of claims it paid. They assert that CMS should recognize proportionality in these situations and likewise proportionally reduce Medicare's demand amount in these cases. NGHP stakeholders stated that if CMS does not proportionally reduce Medicare's demand amount in these situations, it could leave beneficiaries without any compensation for issues such as pain and suffering or lost wages. However, CMS officials said that the concept of proportionality is in conflict with MSP provisions granting CMS a priority right of recovery, which entitles Medicare to full recovery for the expenses it paid up to the settlement amount. Nonetheless, CMS officials said that Medicare beneficiaries may contact the appropriate CMS regional office prior to settling a case to request a pre-demand compromise in the event that the demand amount would consume the entire settlement. CMS officials told us that they do not, however, advertise the availability of this option and do not keep data on how often compromises are requested or granted. Limited MSPRC data on those compromise requests of which the MSPRC is made aware suggest that about two out of every three compromise requests are approved by the reviewing CMS regional office.

---

[32]CMS will not seek recovery of lump sum liability settlements of $300 or less that meet certain criteria—if the beneficiary's settlement is related to an alleged physical-trauma-based incident, the liability insurance (including self-insurance) settlement is for $300 or less, the beneficiary has not yet received and does not expect to receive any other payments related to the incident, and the MSPRC has not previously issued a recovery demand letter.

CMS Is Taking Steps to Address Some Key Challenges We Identified with Aspects of Mandatory Reporting

Determining Whether Individuals Are Medicare Beneficiaries

We identified three key challenges related to aspects of mandatory reporting for NGHPs: determining whether individuals are Medicare beneficiaries, supplying diagnostic codes related to individuals' injuries, and reporting all settlement amounts. CMS reported that it is taking steps to address some, but not all, of these challenges.

NGHP stakeholders reported difficulty in determining whether individuals are Medicare beneficiaries for the purposes of mandatory reporting, and CMS has taken a step to address the challenge and is considering another. NGHP stakeholders have reported difficulty obtaining the information needed from individuals involved in NGHP situations in order to determine whether an individual is a Medicare beneficiary, and whether the NGHP is therefore required to report the situation. In order to verify an individual's Medicare eligibility, an NGHP either needs the person's Medicare Health Insurance Claim Number (HICN) or the person's Social Security number, first initial of the first name and last six characters of the last name, date of birth, and gender. NGHP stakeholders report that individuals are reluctant to surrender sensitive information, such as Social Security numbers, to NGHPs—particularly as there may be an adversarial relationship between the individual and the NGHP (i.e., that individual is suing the insurer or self-insured company). Without this information, the NGHP cannot verify whether the individual is a Medicare beneficiary and cannot submit the mandatory reporting record. Therefore, NGHP stakeholders also reported concerns that they could be subject to mandatory reporting noncompliance fines if not being able to obtain this information led to being unable to submit a mandatory reporting record.[33]

To assist NGHPs with this challenge, CMS has provided them with model language that they can use to document their unsuccessful attempts to obtain individuals' HICNs or Social Security numbers. This model language is a sample statement to be signed by the individual indicating whether the individual is a Medicare beneficiary for use in cases when the NGHPs cannot otherwise determine the individual's Medicare status. CMS has stated that if an individual refuses to furnish a HICN or Social Security number, and the NGHP reporting entity chooses to use this model language, CMS will generally consider the reporting entity

---

[33]As of January 2012, CMS had not yet begun assessing these fines.

compliant for purposes of mandatory reporting.[34] In addition, CMS officials stated that CMS and a number of other federal agencies are currently conducting internal studies to evaluate possible alternatives that could be used in lieu of Social Security numbers.

Supplying Diagnostic Codes

Liability insurance representatives maintain that it is difficult for them to obtain the diagnostic information that CMS requires they report, and CMS officials told us that they were not considering eliminating any of the required data elements for mandatory reporting in the near future. Under mandatory reporting, NGHPs are required to report the International Classification of Diseases, Ninth Revision, Clinical Modification (ICD-9) diagnostic codes related to the claimant's injury. However, liability insurers have historically not had access to such detailed information about a claimant's injuries, and they report difficulty in obtaining these codes.[35] Prior to January 1, 2011, CMS allowed NGHPs to submit a text description of an individual's injury in lieu of ICD-9 codes, but the text description is no longer allowed. Without ICD-9 codes, liability insurers are unable to submit a mandatory reporting record. CMS officials told us that NGHPs, including liability insurers, should be able to obtain ICD-9 codes for the purposes of reporting. For example, they said that beneficiaries and their attorneys know the claims involved in their particular MSP situations and could share the claims with the NGHP. However, while this information is required to be reported, CMS may already have this information if the agency has already been notified of the MSP situation because the codes are required to create an MSP record within the CMS data systems. MSPRC officials told us that CMS was already aware of the MSP situations for about 90 percent of cases currently reported via mandatory reporting because MSP records were

---

[34]CMS will consider the reporting entity compliant for purposes of mandatory reporting if a signed copy of the model language is obtained and retained (even if the individual is later discovered to be a Medicare beneficiary). With respect to cases where ongoing responsibility for medical items and services applies, CMS suggests that the model language be re-signed and dated at least once every 12 months and kept available on file by the NGHP. CMS notes that this process does not provide a "safe harbor" to any reporting entity attempting to use it to avoid reporting MSP data about an individual known to the reporting entity to be a Medicare beneficiary.

[35]ICD-9 codes are used by the Medicare claims contractors to determine whether specific Medicare claims should be denied or paid. NGHPs submitting incorrect ICD-9 codes could result in beneficiaries' claims that are actually unrelated to their MSP situations being incorrectly denied.

created within the CMS data systems. Therefore, CMS would already have had access to the related codes.

Reporting on All Settlements

Some NGHP stakeholders assert that they should not have to report all liability settlements, as CMS may be able to recover very little from certain settlements,[36] and CMS is evaluating data to determine if appropriate reporting thresholds could be established. An official of an organization representing NGHPs has stated that liability settlements of less than $25,000 include a small portion of annual settlement payments but constitute a large number of individual claims. Therefore, the official suggested that liability NGHPs should not have to report these settlements to CMS as it would just increase the reporting burden on NGHPs while yielding small recovery amounts. However, recovery data show that for fiscal year 2011, the MSPRC issued almost 57,000 demands for liability settlements under $25,000. These demands related to these settlements totaled almost $71 million, with an average demand amount of about $1,250.

Nonetheless, CMS is evaluating its data and the agency is considering implementing reporting thresholds, if appropriate. However, CMS officials expressed concern that setting reporting thresholds could have unintended consequences. If thresholds were set at, for example, $25,000, then the NGHP industry might begin settling many cases at amounts just under $25,000 in order to avoid mandatory reporting. CMS officials reported that any determination of reporting thresholds should wait until liability reporting data are available so the data can be analyzed and an appropriate threshold set. CMS officials also note that the establishment of any mandatory reporting thresholds would not eliminate CMS's recovery rights for settlements below the threshold.

---

[36]Not all liability settlements are currently required to be reported, and there is a phased-in schedule for liability reporting based on the total settlement amount. However, all settlements "over minimum threshold" are scheduled to begin reporting on January 1, 2013. The current minimum reporting threshold is $5,000 for liability settlements with no ongoing responsibility for medical items and services. That threshold is currently scheduled to decrease over time and eventually will be eliminated.

CMS Has Taken Few Steps to Address Challenges Related to Insufficient and Confusing CMS Guidance and Communication about NGHP MSP Situations

We identified key challenges related to CMS guidance and communication of information on the MSP process, guidance on MSAs, and beneficiary rights and responsibilities related to MSP recoveries, resulting in communication of information that does not meet GAO standards for internal control. CMS has taken few steps to address these challenges.

Overall MSP Process Guidance on the CMS Website

The overall presentation and organization of MSP process guidance for situations involving NGHPs on the CMS website does not ensure that pertinent information can be identified by external stakeholders, including NGHPs. For example, there is no main web page for the MSP program. Instead, information relevant to the MSP process for situations involving NGHPs is categorized on the main Medicare home page in two separate sections—some MSP process information falls under "Coordination of Benefits" and other process information falls under "Medicare Secondary Payer Recovery." This makes it difficult to find any recent developments or changes to the MSP process as a whole, as an individual has to check multiple web pages to locate recent news. Additionally, while CMS has created an MSP manual, there is no direct link to the manual under the Coordination of Benefits or Medicare Secondary Payer Recovery headings on the Medicare home page. Also, because CMS regularly updates its MSP policies and process by issuing memos or "alerts," it is difficult to determine what the current policy is or what may have changed in the process.

CMS Guidance regarding MSAs

CMS has issued guidance regarding WCMSAs, but finding current, official WCMSA guidance can be challenging, and CMS has issued little other MSA guidance. While CMS has a policy manual for describing the MSP process in general, no similar manual, or chapter in the MSP process policy manual, describes WCMSA policy. Further, while guidance in the form of memorandums related to WCMSAs exists, no manual or similar document currently exists to organize this guidance. The WCMSA-related memorandums are accessible on the CMS website, but are poorly organized, making it difficult to find memorandums on particular topics. As a result, NGHP stakeholders have reported that it is difficult to find updated WCMSA policies. However, CMS officials told us in January 2012 that the agency was developing a WCMSA user manual that would be available through the CMS website. Stakeholders also said that the WCMSA review and approval criteria are not clear, and expressed a desire for CMS to make this information more transparent. Furthermore, CMS has established an e-mail address to accept questions regarding

WCMSA submission policy, but the actual e-mail address is not well publicized and is difficult to find.

Additionally, while guidance exists for WCMSAs, CMS has issued very little guidance related to liability MSAs and NGHP stakeholders reported inconsistent handling of liability MSAs. CMS issued its first formal memorandum related to MSA for liability situations on September 29, 2011, detailing when it would consider Medicare's interests satisfied with respect to future medical expenses in liability settlements.[37] But this is the only formal memorandum related to liability MSAs that CMS has provided. And unlike for WCMSAs, CMS does not have a formal review and approval process for liability or no-fault MSA arrangements. Upon request, some CMS regional offices will review liability or no-fault MSAs, but this is at the regional office's discretion. NGHP stakeholders report variation in regional office response, including which regional offices will review liability MSAs, policies (such as setting thresholds for review), and regional office responsiveness. Regarding developing policies and procedures for liability MSAs, CMS officials report that the agency is working to operationalize policy regarding the reporting of future medical expenses in liability insurance situations, including an option to allow for an immediate payment to Medicare for future medical costs. This would provide an additional option for taking Medicare's interests into account rather than the option of establishing an MSA. CMS officials did not report that they were taking any steps to address regional office variation in liability MSA review.

CMS Communications with Beneficiaries

CMS communications with beneficiaries regarding their rights and responsibilities in the MSP recovery process are not always sufficient or clear and CMS has taken few steps to address this challenge. Specifically, two letters sent to beneficiaries are not sufficient or clear with regard to the beneficiary's rights to dispute unrelated claims. The rights and responsibilities letter, which is sent to beneficiaries by the MSPRC after it is notified of an MSP situation, does not make beneficiaries' rights and responsibilities clear regarding their ability to dispute the conditional payments that the MSPRC identifies. While the letter notes that the

---

[37]CMS clarified that if the beneficiary's treating physician certifies in writing that treatment for the alleged injury related to the liability insurance settlement has been completed as of the date of the settlement, and that future medical items and services for that injury will not be required, Medicare considers its interests satisfied with respect to future medical items and services for the settlement.

beneficiary should expect to receive a letter detailing the conditional payments Medicare has made to date, it does not explain that this letter may contain some unrelated claims and the beneficiary should review the document carefully. Furthermore, it does not explain that the beneficiary has the right to dispute any claims unrelated to the MSP situation. While CMS revised the rights and responsibilities letter in 2011, the revisions did not address these issues.[38]

Beneficiaries also receive a conditional payment letter, which CMS regards as a first step in determining conditional payments, but that is not made clear to the beneficiaries. Beneficiary advocates report that these letters often include charges for unrelated medical services. As a consequence, according to an attorney who represents Medicare beneficiaries, beneficiaries are often asked to return too great a portion of their settlements to Medicare. CMS officials stated that they consider the conditional payment letter the first attempt at determining the conditional payments based on the information the MSPRC has, and that they want the beneficiary and beneficiary's attorney to help clarify which claims are related. They told us that the beneficiary is in the best position to clarify which claims are related, and that the MSPRC will work with the beneficiary and the beneficiary's attorney prior to issuing the demand letter. However, while the conditional payment letter states that the beneficiary should inform the MSPRC if any of the identified conditional payments are inaccurate or incomplete, the language used in the conditional payment letter does not convey that the MSPRC will work with the beneficiary and the beneficiary's attorney prior to issuing the demand letter. Additionally, the letter does not include that CMS may be willing to compromise its demand amount if it appears the conditional payments will consume the beneficiary's entire settlement. The letter also does not include the beneficiary's rights to appeal the amount of the MSP claim, as well as to seek a waiver of recovery, once the demand letter is issued. CMS did not report any plans to revise the language used in the conditional payment letter.

---

[38]CMS revised the rights and responsibilities letter by omitting a statement that Medicare should be repaid before funds disbursed for other purposes. The agency also added a statement that Medicare will not take any collection action if an appeal or waiver is pending.

Conclusions

CMS has a responsibility to protect the Medicare Trust Funds by ensuring that funds owed the program are recovered. Mandatory reporting should increase CMS's awareness of MSP situations and therefore increase recoveries and MSP savings. Thus far, the initial implementation of mandatory reporting for NGHPs has greatly increased the number of MSP NGHP situations reported to CMS. MSP savings have also shown increases and should continue to increase as mandatory reporting is fully implemented. However, the volume of liability settlements that have yet to be reported to CMS is unknown; therefore, the extent to which workloads, recoveries, and savings will increase is also unknown.

As a result of mandatory reporting, some NGHPs, particularly liability insurers, are interacting with CMS for the first time. Some of these NGHPs and NGHP stakeholder groups have raised concerns about long-standing MSP process and policies. Additionally, mandatory reporting increased the MSP contractors' workloads, leading to performance delays. CMS has been responsive to some of the concerns expressed by NGHPs, in particular by continuing to delay the start of mandatory reporting for various types of liability settlements. CMS has also evaluated and modified some of its long-standing MSP policies and procedures, and is in the process of considering additional changes and program improvements. However, because these changes are new or still being implemented, it is too soon to tell the effect that they will have on improving the MSP process. Additionally, there are several areas related to the MSP program and process that still need improvement.

In order to maximize its ability to protect the Medicare Trust Funds, CMS's efforts to recover conditional payments when Medicare should not have been the primary payer need to be cost-effective. CMS recently implemented two recovery thresholds—a low, across-the-board threshold based in part on provisions in the Federal Claims Collection Act and a higher threshold that applies to certain liability MSP situations. CMS officials said the agency will consider setting additional recovery thresholds for certain NGHP situations once the agency has had a chance to review 2012 data. If recovery thresholds need to later be adjusted based on 2012 data, then CMS could make adjustments as appropriate. CMS could also improve program effectiveness by aligning mandatory reporting thresholds with recovery thresholds, once they are set.

Additionally, CMS has opportunities to improve the MSP program by reducing specific reporting requirements for NGHPs and improving communication with stakeholders. While CMS's main goal with mandatory reporting should be to obtain necessary information to pursue MSP recoveries, CMS could take steps to lessen the burden on NGHPs, without substantially increasing the burden on CMS or its contractors. Communication between CMS and various NGHP stakeholders, including beneficiaries, also needs improvement. Ensuring that these stakeholders have current, complete information so that they can understand the MSP process and policies, and their roles and responsibilities in the process, is essential for ensuring the overall effectiveness of the program.

Recommendations for Executive Action

We are making five recommendations to CMS to improve the effectiveness of the MSP program and process for NGHPs.

To ensure cost-effectiveness in the agency's NGHP recovery process, we recommend that the Acting Administrator of CMS review recovery thresholds periodically for appropriateness to ensure that the agency's recovery efforts are being conducted in the most cost-effective manner possible, and not require NGHPs to report on cases for which the agency will not seek any recovery.

To potentially decrease the administrative burden of mandatory reporting for NGHPs, we recommend that the Acting Administrator of CMS consider making the submission of ICD-9 codes an optional component of reporting for liability NGHPs.

To improve the agency's communication regarding the MSP process for situations involving NGHPs. we recommend that the Acting Administrator of CMS take the following three actions:

- develop a centralized MSP program website, to include links to information about the various parts of the MSP process;

- develop guidance regarding liability and no-fault set-aside arrangements; and

- review and revise the correspondence with beneficiaries, such as letters sent during the recovery process, to ensure that beneficiary rights and responsibilities are more clearly communicated.

Agency Comments

We received written comments on a draft of this report from the Department of Health and Human Services on behalf of CMS. These comments are reprinted in appendix I.

CMS agreed with our recommendation to review recovery thresholds periodically for appropriateness and our three recommendations to improve the agency's communication regarding the MSP process for situations involving NGHPs. CMS also agreed to consider our recommendation on potentially making the submission of ICD-9 codes an optional component of reporting for liability NGHPs. However, the agency also noted that about 95 percent of NGHPs reporting data to CMS have provided the required ICD-9 codes, and provided reasons why allowing text descriptions rather than ICD-9 codes could increase the burden on parties such as beneficiaries.

As agreed with your office, unless you publicly announce the contents of this report earlier, we plan no further distribution until 30 days from the report date. At that time, we will send copies to the Secretary of Health and Human Services, the Acting Administrator of CMS, appropriate congressional committees, and other interested parties. In addition, the report will be available at no charge on the GAO website at http://www.gao.gov.

If you or your staff have any questions about this report, please contact me at (202) 512-7114 or kingk@gao.gov. Contact points for our Offices of Congressional Relations and Public Affairs may be found on the last page of this report. GAO staff who made major contributions to this report are listed in appendix II.

Sincerely yours,

Kathleen M. King
Director, Health Care

Appendix I: Comments from the Department of Health and Human Services

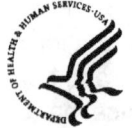

DEPARTMENT OF HEALTH & HUMAN SERVICES   OFFICE OF THE SECRETARY

Assistant Secretary for Legislation
Washington, DC 20201

FEB 27 2012

Kathleen King
Director, Health Care
U.S. Government Accountability Office
441 G Street NW
Washington, DC 20548

Dear Ms. King:

Attached are comments on the U.S. Government Accountability Office's (GAO) report entitled, "MEDICARE SECONDARY PAYER: Additional Steps Are Needed to Improve Program Effectiveness for Non-Group Health Plans" (GAO-12-333).

The Department appreciates the opportunity to review this draft section of the report prior to publication.

Sincerely,

Jim R. Esquea
Assistant Secretary for Legislation

Attachment

GENERAL COMMENTS OF THE DEPARTMENT OF HEALTH AND HUMAN SERVICES (HHS) ON THE GOVERNMENT ACCOUNTABILITY OFFICE'S (GAO) DRAFT REPORT ENTITLED, "MEDICARE SECONDARY PAYER: ADDITIONAL STEPS ARE NEEDED TO IMPROVE PROGRAM EFFECTIVENESS FOR NON-GROUP HEALTH PLANS" (GAO-12-333)

GAO Recommendation

To ensure cost-effectiveness in the agency's Non-Group Health Plans (NGHPs) recovery process, we recommend that the Acting Administrator of CMS review recovery thresholds periodically for appropriateness to ensure that the agency's recovery efforts are being conducted in the most cost-effective manner possible, and not require NGHPs to report on cases for which the agency will not seek any recovery.

CMS Response

The CMS concurs with this recommendation. The CMS has already implemented two recovery thresholds and is considering other additional recovery thresholds. The CMS will continue to monitor and evaluate the data received via Section 111 reporting to determine if these thresholds should be adjusted and whether additional recovery thresholds can be implemented to achieve cost-effective processes. Any new recovery thresholds must balance protecting Medicare's interests with NGHP stakeholder's concerns.

GAO Recommendation

To potentially decrease the administrative burden of mandatory reporting for NGHPs, we recommend that the Acting Administrator of CMS consider making the submission of ICD-9 codes an optional component of reporting for liability NGHPs.

CMS Response

The CMS will consider this recommendation. It is important to note that the International Classification of Diseases, Ninth Revision (ICD-9) codes are the national standard identifiers used to classify health care diagnoses. These codes are recorded on the beneficiary's medical care statements/bills. The NGHPs routinely obtain the codes from the beneficiary or starting with a textual description of the diagnosis may obtain ICD-9 coding reference materials to assign the diagnosis codes. A link to a complete listing of ICD-9 codes is also available from the Section 111 NGHP User Guide. While there was initial concern by some NGHPs regarding the supplying of ICD-9 codes as part of the Section 111 mandatory reporting process, many NGHPs have successfully used them. As of January 2012, CMS has received files from over 14,000 NGHP insurers containing the required ICD-9 codes. This figure represents approximately 95 percent of NGHPs reporting data to CMS.

To assist those that still need help setting up their reporting process to include ICD-9 codes, CMS has provided considerable educational materials to industry. This includes free computer-based training modules and assistance from technical representatives assigned to insurers by the Coordination of Benefits Contractor. We believe these efforts have been successful because we now receive very few questions or complaints from NGHPs regarding the use of ICD-9 codes.

GENERAL COMMENTS OF THE DEPARTMENT OF HEALTH AND HUMAN SERVICES (HHS) ON THE GOVERNMENT ACCOUNTABILITY OFFICE'S (GAO) DRAFT REPORT ENTITLED, "MEDICARE SECONDARY PAYER: ADDITIONAL STEPS ARE NEEDED TO IMPROVE PROGRAM EFFECTIVENESS FOR NON-GROUP HEALTH PLANS" (GAO-12-333)

The ICD-9 codes are the most reliable way to identify the actual claims related to an incident where there was a settlement. Since these codes are standard they allow for a one to one match of claims paid to the claims that relate to the incident under settlement. If CMS allowed text descriptions rather than ICD-9 codes, this would increase the burden on all parties including providers and beneficiaries for the following reasons:

- The vast majority of health care data is processed electronically, and code sets represent the most efficient way for entities to gather, process and consistently disseminate large volumes of data in a universally recognized format.

- Text information about treatment could lead to inconsistent information and could require more manual follow-up.

- Eliminating the reporting of ICD-9 codes could lead to an increase in inappropriately denied claims, and incorrect demands to beneficiaries.

GAO Recommendation

To improve the agency's communication regarding the MSP process for situations involving NGHPs, we recommend that the Acting Administrator develop a centralized MSP program website to include links to information about various parts of the MSP process.

CMS Response

The CMS concurs with this recommendation and is actively working to consolidate MSP information. The consolidation of MSP information is central to CMS' new contacting strategy. This new strategy includes one central point of contact for CMS stakeholders and one single website for all aspects of MSP policy and operations.

GAO Recommendation

To improve the agency's communication regarding the MSP process for situations involving NGHPs, we recommend that the Acting Administrator develop guidance regarding liability and no-fault set aside arrangements.

CMS Response

The CMS concurs with this recommendation. The CMS is working to clarify some longstanding liability and no-fault set-aside policy and plans to use notice and comment rulemaking to seek industry comments related to these areas of the MSP program.

**GENERAL COMMENTS OF THE DEPARTMENT OF HEALTH AND HUMAN
SERVICES (HHS) ON THE GOVERNMENT ACCOUNTABILITY OFFICE'S (GAO)
DRAFT REPORT ENTITLED, "MEDICARE SECONDARY PAYER: ADDITIONAL
STEPS ARE NEEDED TO IMPROVE PROGRAM EFFECTIVENESS FOR NON-
GROUP HEALTH PLANS" (GAO-12-333)**

GAO Recommendation

To improve the agency's communication regarding the MSP process for situations involving
NGHPs, we recommend that the Acting Administrator review and revise the correspondence
with beneficiaries, such as letters sent during the recovery process, to ensure that beneficiary
rights and responsibilities are more clearly communicated.

CMS Response

The CMS concurs with this recommendation.   In October 2011, CMS reviewed and revised the
Rights and Responsibilities (RAR) letter, as well as the Conditional Payment Notice (CPN).
These revisions focused on providing beneficiaries with information on the new options
available to them, while focusing on streamlining the legal language so that it is more easily
understood. We used section headings in order to direct the reader to the aspects of the letter that
are most relevant to him or her. We reduced each letter so that it contains exactly what the
reader needs to know at the specified point in the process.

The CMS intends to review all MSP-related correspondence, including the revisions to the
aforementioned letters, and make further revisions as necessary.

Appendix II: GAO Contact and Staff Acknowledgments

GAO Contact	Kathleen M. King, (202) 512-7114 or kingk@gao.gov
Staff Acknowledgments	In addition to the contact named above, key contributors to this report were Gerardine Brennan, Assistant Director; Christina Ritchie; and Lisa Rogers. Laurie Pachter; Jessica C. Smith; and Jennifer Whitworth also provided valuable assistance.

GAO's Mission	The Government Accountability Office, the audit, evaluation, and investigative arm of Congress, exists to support Congress in meeting its constitutional responsibilities and to help improve the performance and accountability of the federal government for the American people. GAO examines the use of public funds; evaluates federal programs and policies; and provides analyses, recommendations, and other assistance to help Congress make informed oversight, policy, and funding decisions. GAO's commitment to good government is reflected in its core values of accountability, integrity, and reliability.
Obtaining Copies of GAO Reports and Testimony	The fastest and easiest way to obtain copies of GAO documents at no cost is through GAO's website (www.gao.gov). Each weekday afternoon, GAO posts on its website newly released reports, testimony, and correspondence. To have GAO e-mail you a list of newly posted products, go to www.gao.gov and select "E-mail Updates."
Order by Phone	The price of each GAO publication reflects GAO's actual cost of production and distribution and depends on the number of pages in the publication and whether the publication is printed in color or black and white. Pricing and ordering information is posted on GAO's website, http://www.gao.gov/ordering.htm. Place orders by calling (202) 512-6000, toll free (866) 801-7077, or TDD (202) 512-2537. Orders may be paid for using American Express, Discover Card, MasterCard, Visa, check, or money order. Call for additional information.
Connect with GAO	Connect with GAO on Facebook, Flickr, Twitter, and YouTube. Subscribe to our RSS Feeds or E-mail Updates. Listen to our Podcasts. Visit GAO on the web at www.gao.gov.
To Report Fraud, Waste, and Abuse in Federal Programs	Contact: Website: www.gao.gov/fraudnet/fraudnet.htm E-mail: fraudnet@gao.gov Automated answering system: (800) 424-5454 or (202) 512-7470
Congressional Relations	Katherine Siggerud, Managing Director, siggerudk@gao.gov, (202) 512-4400, U.S. Government Accountability Office, 441 G Street NW, Room 7125, Washington, DC 20548
Public Affairs	Chuck Young, Managing Director, youngc1@gao.gov, (202) 512-4800 U.S. Government Accountability Office, 441 G Street NW, Room 7149 Washington, DC 20548

Please Print on Recycled Paper.

www.ingramcontent.com/pod-product-compliance
Lightning Source LLC
Chambersburg PA
CBHW080920290526
45795CB00007BA/2591

9 781492 751281